Brain Cancer Awareness

Developing Networks of Strength, Hope, and Healing
Empowering Patients, Caregivers, and Loved Ones with
Innovative Therapies and Groundbreaking Treatments

Michele L. Valdez

Introducing the exclusive and captivating world of Michele L. Valdez. Immerse yourself in the timeless elegance and creativity that defines our brand. Experience the unparalleled craftsmanship and attention to detail that sets us apart. Discover the essence of sophistication and style with our exquisite collection.

T a b l e   o f   C o n t e n t s

Preface

Step into a realm where uncertainty is conquered, where the shadows of illness are banished by a radiant glow. Behold a shining symbol of the indomitable human spirit. Step into the extraordinary world of "Brain Cancer" where every page overflows with stories of bravery, profound knowledge about the latest advancements in treatments, and a guiding path to gracefully and fearlessly navigate the complex maze of brain cancer.

Experience the incredible journey of survivors, brave warriors who have fearlessly confronted the challenging diagnosis of brain cancer. Uncover the awe-inspiring strength of resilience and witness the indomitable human spirit conquering seemingly impossible challenges through their captivating stories. Discover the awe-inspiring power that lies dormant within each and every one of us, ready to be unleashed when confronted with life's greatest challenges. These captivating stories serve as a powerful reminder of the indomitable strength that resides within, just waiting to be awakened.

Step into a realm of extraordinary healing that transcends traditional methods. Discover the harmonious fusion of age-old wisdom and cutting-edge science, meticulously crafted to nourish your mind, restore your body, and bring solace to your soul. Embark on a profound exploration of mindfulness, nutrition, and alternative therapies as we delve into the awe-inspiring world of holistic healing. Discover the extraordinary transformative power it holds in your journey towards recovery.

Experience the awe-inspiring world of medical innovation, where revolutionary treatments and state-of-the-art technologies are transforming the very fabric of brain cancer care. Experience the cutting-edge world of tomorrow's treatments today, as we reveal the future of cancer care and the incredible promise it holds for those seeking hope. Explore the exciting realms of precision medicine and immunotherapy, where groundbreaking advancements are revolutionizing the fight against cancer. Join us on this journey towards a brighter future.

Embark on a fearless expedition through the intricate maze of brain cancer, equipped with invaluable insights and professional recommendations that will empower and enlighten your path. Unlock a treasure trove of wisdom and practical advice to conquer the hurdles of brain cancer with elegance and strength. Explore expert tips on managing treatment side effects and nurturing your emotional well-being. Embrace invaluable insights and actionable strategies to navigate the challenges of brain cancer with grace and resilience.

Discover the transformative power of community - where strength becomes unwavering, healing becomes profound, and thriving becomes inevitable. Embark on a remarkable journey with like-minded adventurers, as we come together to create unbreakable connections and unwavering encouragement that surpass the limitations of illness. Experience the power of unity as we transcend the darkness of despair, joining forces in our unwavering pursuit of healing and a brighter future.

Prepare to embark on a transformative journey as you reach the last page of "Brain Cancer". Let the profound wisdom you have acquired from the pages of this remarkable book become an invaluable companion on your path forward.Introducing the all-new, revolutionary text transformation service! Get ready to experience the power of copywriting magic as we transform your Let it shine as a radiant beacon, illuminating even the darkest of nights. Discover its power as a wellspring of strength during uncertain times. Embrace it as a guiding light on your path to healing, a beacon of hope that never wavers. Discover the extraordinary journey that awaits within the pages of this remarkable book. It is more than just a collection of words; it is a lifeline that will captivate your heart and inspire your soul. Prepare to be moved by the indomitable resilience of the human spirit and the limitless power of hope that permeates every chapter.

Introduction

In a world where new difficulties arise every day, there is one conflict that knows no bounds and unites us all in the fight against brain cancer. Introducing "Brain Cancer Awareness," a ground-breaking book that raises awareness of one of the most urgent health issues of our day. This book is more than just a call to action—it's a beacon of hope in the dark, a rallying cry for change, and a tribute to the strength of group action in the face of adversity—thanks to its captivating storylines, knowledgeable insights, and doable solutions.

This handbook invites readers to delve into the centre of the problem, where the harsh facts of brain cancer are revealed. Readers are given a fuller knowledge of the impact of this dreadful disease on individuals, families, and communities worldwide through the emotional stories of survival, loss, and perseverance. This guide acts as a wake-up call, inspiring readers to take up the battle against brain cancer with its startling facts and personal stories of those impacted.

Since knowledge is power, readers now have the knowledge necessary to comprehend the nuances of brain cancer. This guide offers a thorough overview of the science underlying brain cancer, including everything from the biology of the condition to the most recent developments in research and treatment. Leading oncologists, researchers, and advocates provide expert insights that clarify diagnosis intricacies, treatment options, and the ongoing search for a solution. This information equips readers to become knowledgeable change agents in their own communities.

The idea that "knowledge begets responsibility" motivates readers to take up the cause of brain cancer prevention. This article examines the various methods that individuals may improve the lives of persons affected by brain cancer, ranging from local activism to international advocacy campaigns. Readers are invited to discover their own special methods of supporting the cause and acting as a catalyst for good in the world, be it by increasing awareness, generating money for research, or offering assistance to patients and caregivers.

Readers are reminded that despite hardship, there is always cause for optimism in the midst of the gloom cast by brain cancer. This guide honors the human spirit and the ability of hope to illuminate the path ahead through tales of resiliency, bravery, and victory. Readers learn that there is hope for those impacted by brain cancer through cutting-edge therapies and ground-breaking treatments, encouraging them to never give up on the hope of a better tomorrow.

After reading this book, readers will have a stronger sense of purpose, a stronger sense of dedication to the cause, and a strong desire to improve the lives of individuals who are afflicted by brain cancer. They went forth into the world, unified in their mission to raise awareness, empower minds, and save lives, with knowledge as their guide and hope as their compass. Because every voice matters, every action counts, and when we band together, we can make a difference in the fight against brain cancer.

Join the worldwide effort to save lives, empower minds, and increase awareness. Get a copy of "Brain Cancer Awareness" now and help combat one of the most important health issues of our day. If we work together, we can change things. When we get together, individuals impacted by brain cancer can find hope. We can alter the world if we work together.

Chapter 1

What does brain cancer mean?

Brain cancers develop due to unusual cell growth within the brain. Brain fatalities can result from damage to primary brain cells, other brain components like membranes and arteries, or the spread of malignant cells from other organs to the brain through the bloodstream (metastatic or secondary brain tumor).

Not all brain growths are cancerous, even though they are commonly referred to as brain tumors. Cancer is just a group of cells. A benign tumor is made up of non-cancerous cells. A malignant tumor consists of cancer cells. Malignancy refers specifically to malignant tumors. Cancerous growths consist of rapidly multiplying, distorted cells referred to as cancer cells.

Malignant tumors aggressively spread and invade healthy cells, overpowering them by taking over their space, bloodstream, and nutrients. Similar to all cells in your body, tumor cells require blood and nutrients to stay alive. This issue is particularly problematic in the brain, where increased growth within the limited space of the skull can lead to elevated pressure inside the head (intracranial pressure) or the misalignment of brain regions, impacting their proper function. Both malignant and benign brain tumors can lead to increased intracranial pressure and its consequences. Malignant brain tumors typically lead to these issues more aggressively and rapidly compared to benign brain tumors.

Almost all brain tumors do not metastasize to other parts of the body. One notable distinction between benign and malignant tumors is that benign cysts tend to grow alongside neighboring cells without invading them, unlike malignant tumors which can rapidly invade brain tissues.

Typically, a benign tumor is less serious than a malignant tumor. Nevertheless, a benign tumor can still lead to various complications in the brain, although typically, the symptoms improve at a slower pace compared to malignant tumors (such as in the case of Hippel-Lindau disease, which can affect both benign and malignant tumors in the Central Nervous System).

Brain aneurysms are occasionally mistaken for brain tumors. Brain aneurysms are not tumors. They can be weak areas in the brain arteries or blood vessels that expand and form a ballooning or growth in the vessel wall. Usually, there are no noticeable symptoms unless they begin to leak blood into the surrounding brain tissues or if they rupture. Aneurysms can be present at birth or develop in brain vessels due to vessel damage, such as stress, atherosclerosis, or high blood pressure, but they do not originate from cancer cells. Unfortunately, when aneurysms present symptoms, they may mimic those caused by brain tumors. Spinal cord tumors such as chordomas and other malignancies or attacks in tissues near the brain can cause symptoms similar to those seen in primary and secondary brain tumors

Our bodies contain a multitude of cells that continuously grow and multiply to support our natural bodily processes. When brain cells deviate from their normal development process, instead of fixing damage, they can actually end up causing it. When these unusual brain cells start to proliferate within the brain, they can lead to the development of a brain tumor. Rapid cell development within the brain can result in the need for a brain tumor diagnosis.

If cells fail in another part of the body, such as the lungs, and then spread to the brain, it is known as secondary brain cancer or metastases.

Chapter 2

Brain Cancer: Understanding the Root Causes

Brain tumors originating in the brain:

- Neuralgia auditory

- Schwannoma (acoustic neuroma).

Brain tumors typically develop within the brain or nearby structures like the meninges, cranial nerves, pituitary gland, or pineal gland.

Brain tumors typically begin when normal cells develop mutations in their DNA. These mutations enable cells to proliferate and survive beyond the normal lifespan of healthy cells. This results in numerous abnormal cells that come together to create a tumor.

Primary brain tumors in adults are much less frequent

compared to secondary brain tumors, which originate in other parts of the body and then spread to the brain.

There are various primary brain tumors. Every name is derived from the specific type of cells it encompasses. For instance:

Gliomas are tumors that originate in the brain or spinal cord. A variety of brain tumors are astrocytomas, ependymomas, glioblastomas, oligoastrocytomas, and oligodendrogliomas.

Originating from the membranes surrounding the brain and spinal cord, meningiomas are tumors worth noting. Typically, meningiomas are benign.

Acoustic neuromas, also known as schwannomas, are non-cancerous growths that form on the nerves responsible for balance and hearing, connecting the inner ear to the brain.

Pituitary adenomas are typically benign growths that form in the pituitary gland located at the base of the brain. These tumors have a significant impact on the human pituitary hormones, which in turn affect the entire body.

Medulloblastomas are the most common malignant brain tumors found in children. A medulloblastoma originates in the lower back region of the brain and can spread through the cerebrospinal fluid. These tumors are not as frequently seen in adults.

During childhood, germ cell tumors can develop in the area where the testicles or ovaries will form. Occasionally, germ cell tumors can impact different parts of your body, such as the brain.

Craniopharyngiomas are rare, benign growths that develop near the pituitary gland in the brain, responsible for regulating various bodily functions through hormone secretion. As the craniopharyngioma slowly expands, it disrupts the pituitary gland and other structures near the brain.

Cancer originating in another part of the body and spreading to the brain:

Brain tumors that develop from cancers originating in

other parts of the body and then spread to the brain are known as supplementary (metastatic) brain tumors.

Additional brain tumors often develop in people with a previous cancer diagnosis. Occasionally, a metastatic brain tumor may be the initial sign of a cancer that originated elsewhere in the body.

Supplementary brain tumors are more frequently observed in adults compared to primary brain tumors.

Tumors have the potential to spread to the brain, with some common types being:

- Breast cancer

- Malignancy of the colon

- Kidney cancer

- Lung cancer

- Melanoma.

Factors that Contribute to Brain Cancer

The cause of principal brain tumors in most individuals remains unknown. Doctors have identified certain factors that could increase your risk of developing a brain tumor.

Factors that increase the likelihood of risk are:

- Being exposed to ionizing radiations increases the risk of brain tumors. There are different types of ionizing rays such as those used in cancer treatment and exposure from atomic bombs.

- Brain tumors can sometimes be traced back to a family history of the condition or genetic syndromes that increase the risk.

Brain Tumor Diagnosis

If a brain tumor is suspected, your doctor may suggest various tests and procedures, such as:

During a neurological examination, various activities are performed to assess your eyesight, hearing, balance, coordination, strength, and reflexes. Struggles in one or multiple areas could indicate the specific part of the brain affected by a brain tumor.

When it comes to imaging assessments, Magnetic Resonance Imaging (MRI) is frequently utilized in the diagnosis of brain tumors. At times, a dye might be injected into a vein in your arm during your MRI evaluation.

Your doctor can utilize various MRI scan components such as functional MRI, perfusion MRI, and magnetic resonance spectroscopy to assess the tumor and determine the appropriate treatment.

At times, additional imaging tests may be suggested, such as Computerized Tomography (CT). Positron emission tomography can also be used for brain imaging, although it is generally less effective for visualizing brain tumors compared to other types of cancer.

Evaluations for Detecting Tumors in Different Body Regions

If a human brain tumor is suspected to have originated from cancer in another part of the body, your doctor may suggest tests and procedures to identify the primary cancer source. One option is a CT scan to investigate signs of lung cancer.

Gathering and evaluating a sample of abnormal cells (biopsy):

One option is to perform a biopsy during surgery to remove the brain tumor, or it can be done using a needle.

For brain tumors, a stereotactic needle biopsy can reach delicate areas in the brain without the need for more invasive surgery. A small hole is drilled into the skull by your neurosurgeon. Next, a slender needle is inserted through the opening. Cells are extracted with a needle guided by CT or MRI scanning.

Examining the biopsy sample under a microscope helps identify whether it is cancerous or benign. Advanced laboratory tests offer valuable insights for your doctor regarding your prognosis and treatment possibilities.

Mayo Clinic utilizes various diagnostic techniques, along with cutting-edge imaging technology such as a high-powered (7-tesla) MRI scanner and Magnetic Resonance Elastography (MRE).

MRE is evaluating the tumor's texture to assist the neurosurgeon in planning its removal more effectively.

Developed by a physician-scientist at the Mayo Center. The Mayo Medical clinic brain tumor team utilizes molecular diagnostics, a personalized medical approach that examines the DNA of the tumor. This genetic test assists doctors in predicting the effectiveness of treatment plans for specific types of brain tumors.

Mayo Clinic's brain tumor team utilizes thorough and accurate diagnostic methods to help your neurosurgeon plan your procedure effectively and reduce the chances of requiring additional surgery.

Therapy

The treatment for a brain tumor is determined by the type, size, and location of the tumor, as well as your general health and personal preferences.

Operation

If the brain tumor is located in a surgically accessible area, the surgeon will strive to remove as much of it as possible.

At times, tumors can be small and easily separated from the surrounding brain tissue, allowing for complete surgery. In some cases, tumors are difficult to separate from surrounding tissues or are situated close to sensitive areas in the human brain, posing risks during surgery. Under these conditions, your doctor removes as much of the tumor as is safe.

Removing certain brain tumors can potentially alleviate your symptoms.

Undergoing brain tumor surgery comes with risks like potential sickness and blood loss. The risks you face can vary depending on the location of the tumor in your brain. For instance, operating on the tumor close to the nerves connected to your eye could pose a risk of vision impairment.

Brain Surgery with Minimal Scarring

Neurosurgeons at Mayo Clinic are highly skilled in performing brain surgery. This procedure, available at only a few medical centers in the United States, can provide assistance to individuals who have received a diagnosis of an inoperable brain tumor. The surgical team can safely remove the tumor with minimal risk of severe complications.

Mayo Center's neurosurgeons excel in minimally invasive techniques. People who undergo brain tumor surgery using these advanced techniques typically have fewer complications, shorter recovery periods, and a lower mortality rate. After undergoing brain tumor surgery at Mayo Medical clinic, many individuals aim to leave as soon as they can. Neurosurgeons excel at performing precise and intricate surgeries by collaborating with brain imaging specialists (neuroradiologists) and utilizing state-of-the-art medical navigation and mapping technology. They were able to clearly imagine the location of the tumor and the most effective route to reach it.

Radiation treatment

Rays therapy involves the use of high-energy beams like X-rays or protons to eliminate tumor cells. The therapy involving rays can be administered from a machine outside the body (exterior beam rays) or, in rare cases, the rays can be placed inside the body near the brain tumor (brachytherapy).

Exterior beam radiation can target the specific area of the brain with the tumor or be used for whole-brain radiation. Treating cancer that has spread to the brain from other parts of the body and formed multiple cysts in the mind often involves using whole-brain radiation.

Proton beam therapy, a newer form of radiation treatment, has been researched for treating individuals with brain tumors. When dealing with tumors near sensitive parts of the brain, proton therapy can help reduce the chances of side effects linked to radiation. Proton therapy has not yet surpassed standard radiation therapy using X-rays.

The side effects of radiation therapy vary based on the radiation dose you receive. Typical symptoms following write-offs may include fatigue, headaches, memory loss, and scalp sensitivity.

Specialized treatment using focused radiation beams

Gamma rays are used to provide radiation to the head

Gamma Blade stereotactic radiosurgery

Targeted radiosurgery

Stereotactic radiosurgery is not considered traditional surgery. Radiosurgery involves using multiple beams of radiation to deliver a highly focused treatment to target and destroy tumor cells within a precise area. Every individual beam may not be very strong on its own, but when they all converge at the brain tumor, a significant amount of radiation is delivered to eliminate the tumor cells. Various types of technology are used in radiosurgery to deliver radiation for treating brain tumors, such as the Gamma Knife or linear accelerator.

Radiosurgery is usually completed in a single session, allowing you to return home on the same day.

Chemotherapy

Chemotherapy involves the use of medications to eliminate cancer cells. Chemotherapy medications are available in tablet form for oral consumption or can be administered through a vein. Temozolomide (Temodar) is a common chemotherapy medication for treating brain tumors, typically administered in tablet form. There are numerous chemotherapy drugs available for use depending on the type of cancer.

The side effects of chemotherapy vary based on the type and amount of drugs you receive. Chemotherapy may lead to symptoms such as nausea, vomiting, and hair loss.

Testing human brain tumor cells can help determine if chemotherapy is the best treatment option for you. Identifying the type of brain tumor you have is crucial in determining whether chemotherapy is recommended.

Specialized Treatment for Your Health Needs

Prescription drugs are designed to target specific abnormalities found in cancer cells. Targeted prescription drugs can eliminate tumor cells by blocking these abnormalities.

Specialized drugs are available for specific brain tumor types, with ongoing research in clinical trials for additional options. Various targeted therapies are currently in development.

One treatment after another

Therapeutic conversation

Given the potential impact on essential functions like skills, speech, eyesight, and thinking, treatment is often a crucial component of the recovery process for brain tumors. According to your requirements, your doctor might refer you to:

- Regain lost skills or muscle strength with the help of physical therapy.

- Occupational therapy can help you resume your regular daily activities, such as work, following a brain tumor or other illnesses.

- Therapy sessions with specialists in communication difficulties (speech pathologists) can assist with speech issues.

- Providing educational support for children to navigate shifts in their memory and learning abilities.

Exploring alternative methods of healing

There is limited research available on alternative treatments for brain tumors. There is no evidence that alternative therapies can cure brain tumors. Yet, there are additional treatments available to assist in managing the stress of analyzing the brain tumor.

Here are some additional therapies that can assist you in managing your situation:

- Acupuncture

- Engaging in art therapy

- Engage in physical activity

- Engage in meditation

- Music therapy

- Engage in relaxation exercises.

- Discuss your options with your doctor

Acupuncture treatment

Dealing with challenges and finding assistance

Being diagnosed with a brain tumor can be overwhelming and scary. It might give you the sense of having minimal influence over your health. However, there are ways to cope with the unexpected news and emotions that follow a medical diagnosis. Imagine desiring to:

Get informed about brain tumors to empower yourself in making decisions about your care. Consult your doctor about the specific type of brain tumor you have, your treatment options, and, if desired, your prognosis. Discovering more about brain tumors can help you feel more confident when making treatment choices.

Staying connected with loved ones is crucial for dealing

with a brain tumor. Family and friends can provide valuable assistance, such as helping with household tasks while you're in the hospital. Moreover, they offer psychological assistance when you feel overwhelmed by the circumstances.

Seek out someone to chat with for sure: Find a great listener who is open to hearing you talk about your hopes and worries. This could be a friend or family member. Seeking guidance from a counselor, social worker, clergy member, or cancer support group can also be beneficial.

Consult your doctor for information on local organizations, or refer to your phone directory, library, or cancer organizations such as the National Cancer Institute or the American Cancer Society.

Navigating Your Appointment Successfully

Make sure to book an appointment with your doctor if you notice any symptoms that worry you. When diagnosed with a brain tumor, you may come across various specialists, including:

- Specialists in brain disorders (neurologists)

- Doctors specializing in treating tumors, known as oncologists

- Oncologists who utilize radiation therapy to treat cancer tumors

- Specialists in treating nervous system malignancies, known as neuro-oncologists

- Surgeons specializing in the brain and nervous system (neurosurgeons).

Experts in rehabilitation

Being well-prepared for your visit is a smart choice. Here's a guide to help you prepare and know what to expect during your appointment with the doctor.

Make sure to be aware of any pre-appointment restrictions. When the session is scheduled, you can proceed. Always inquire about any necessary preparations, like dietary restrictions, before proceeding.

Make sure to jot down all the symptoms you're noticing,

even if they seem unrelated to why you scheduled the appointment.

Make sure to write down important personal details, such as any major stressors or recent life events.

Summarize all the medications, vitamins, or supplements you are currently using.

It might be a good idea to bring a relative or friend along. Remembering everything discussed during a scheduled appointment can be quite challenging at times. Someone by your side may remember something you overlooked or forgot.

Make a list of questions to ask your doctor.

Being organized and preparing a list of questions can optimize your time with your physician. Please prioritize your questions based on their importance, in case time is limited. When dealing with a brain tumor, it's important to ask your doctor some fundamental questions:

What type of brain tumor do I have?

Where can I find the location of my brain tumor?

What is the size of my brain tumor?

How severe is my brain tumor?

Is my brain tumor cancerous?

Will I require any extra lab tests?

What are the details of my treatment plans?

Is there any treatment available for my brain tumor?

What are the significant advantages and risks associated with each treatment?

Is there a specific treatment you believe would be most suitable for me?

Is it necessary to consult a specialist? Could you please provide the pricing details?

Is there any printed material available for me to take with me? Which websites would you suggest?

What factors will influence my decision to schedule another appointment?

Along with the questions you have prepared for your doctor, feel free to inquire about any other information you may be curious about.

Anticipating Your Doctor's Actions

Expect to answer numerous questions from your doctor. Being ready to address them can create space for other aspects you wish to manage. Here are some questions your doctor might pose:

- When did your symptoms first begin?

- Have your symptoms been persistent or sporadic?

- How intense are your symptoms?

- What, if anything, occurs to alleviate your symptoms?

- What exacerbates your symptoms, if anything?

Chapter 3

Brain Cancer Varieties

Brain tumors are irregular cell growths in the brain.

Not all brain growths are cancerous, even though they are commonly referred to as brain tumors. A tumor is typically used to refer to malignant growths.

Malignant tumors have a tendency to grow rapidly, dominating healthy cells by seizing their space, bloodstream, and nutrients. They can also spread to distant parts of the body. Similar to all the cells in your body, tumor cells require blood and nutrients to stay alive.

Noncancerous growths that do not spread to nearby tissues or other parts of the body are known as benign tumors.

Typically, a benign tumor is less serious than a malignant tumor. However, a benign tumor can still lead to various issues in the brain by exerting pressure on nearby tissue. Around 6 out of every 1,000 individuals in the U.S. are impacted by brain or nervous system tumors.

Primary Brain Tumors

The brain is made up of various types of cells. Brain fatalities can occur when a certain type of cell deviates from its usual traits. After undergoing alterations, the cells start to grow and divide in unexpected patterns.

As these unique cells develop, they transform into the tumor. Primary brain tumors are named as such because they start in the brain.

Common primary brain tumors include gliomas, meningiomas, pituitary adenomas, vestibular schwannomas, and primitive neuroectodermal tumors (medulloblastomas). Glioma encompasses glioblastomas, astrocytomas, oligodendrogliomas, and ependymomas. Several of these are named after the specific area of the brain or the type of brain cell they originate from.

Metastatic brain cancer

Metastatic brain tumors arise from cancerous cells

originating in another part of the body. Cells migrate to the brain from another tumor through a process known as metastasis. This is a very common type of brain tumor.

Causes of Brain Cancer

Similar to tumors in other parts of the body, the specific cause of most brain cancer is still a mystery. Factors such as genetics, environmental toxins, radiation, HIV infection, and smoking have all been linked to brain cancer. Typically, it's challenging to pinpoint a specific cause.

Symptoms of Brain Cancer

Not all brain tumors display symptoms, and some, like pituitary gland tumors, may go undetected unless a CT scan or MRI is done for a different purpose. Brain malignancy symptoms are broad and not exclusive to brain tumors, suggesting that various other conditions could also cause them. To truly uncover the root cause of the symptoms, undergoing diagnostic testing is essential. Symptoms may arise due to a tumor pressing on or encroaching on other areas of the brain, disrupting their normal function.

Brain swelling can be caused by a tumor or surrounding inflammation.

Primary and metastatic brain cancers share similar symptoms.

Here are the common symptoms:

- Experiencing a headache, weakness, clumsiness, and difficulty walking.

- Experiencing seizures

There is no text to rewrite. Additional vague indicators and signs consist of the following:

- Changes in mental status such as concentration, memory, attention, or alertness

- Nausea and vomiting

- Vision abnormalities

- Speech difficulties

Evolution in cognitive abilities or emotional reactions.

For many individuals, the symptoms of a brain tumor can develop slowly and may go unnoticed by both the affected person and their family. At times, these symptoms may appear more quickly. At times, the individual behaves as if they're experiencing a heat stroke.

When is it necessary to seek medical attention?

If you experience unexplained, prolonged vomiting, it's important to seek medical help immediately.

Experiencing double vision or unexplained blurring of vision, particularly on one side.

Feeling tired or more sleepy than usual.

Experiencing new seizures.

Introducing a fresh type of headaches.

Headaches are a common symptom of brain cancer, but they may not appear until the condition has progressed. If there's a notable shift in your headache patterns, your healthcare provider might recommend visiting a medical facility.

If you have a confirmed brain tumor, it's important to report any new symptoms or sudden worsening of symptoms to the nearest medical center emergency department. Keep an eye out for any additional symptoms that may arise.

Experiencing seizures

- Mental shifts like increased drowsiness, memory issues, or difficulty focusing

- Observable alterations or sensory issues

Struggling with conversation or expressing thoughts, alterations in behavior or personality, coordination issues or trouble walking, nausea/vomiting (particularly in middle-aged or elderly individuals), abrupt fever onset, especially post-chemotherapy.

Brain Cancer Diagnosis

Based on the medical interview and physical examination, it is probable that your medical provider will suspect issues related to the brain or brain stem.

Typically, a CT scan of the brain will be conducted. This examination is akin to an X-ray but provides more intricate information in three different dimensions. Typically, a contrast dye is injected into the bloodstream to detect any irregularities on the scan.

Recently, the MRI scan is often preferred over a CT scan for suspected brain tumors. MRI is highly sensitive in detecting cancer and any related changes. Yet, the majority of organizations continue to rely on the CT scan as the initial diagnostic test.

Individuals with brain cancer often experience additional medical issues, leading to the need for routine tests. These include an assessment of blood, electrolytes, and liver function tests.

If there has been a noticeable change in your mental status, blood or urine tests may be conducted to detect drug use.

If your scans reveal a cancerous brain tumor, you will be

directed to a cancer specialist known as an Oncologist. When someone enters your vicinity, you should be recognized as a specialist in brain tumors, known as a neuro-oncologist.

Confirming the presence of cancer typically involves taking a sample of the tumor for testing. This procedure is known as a biopsy.

One of the most effective methods for locating a biopsy is through surgery. The skull is typically opened to completely remove the tumor, if feasible. A sample is taken from the tumor for further examination.

If the doctor encounters difficulty in extracting the entire tumor, they may only be able to remove a portion of it.

There are cases where a biopsy can be obtained without the need to open the skull. The specific location of the tumor in the brain is determined by using a CT or MRI scan. An incision is made in the head, allowing a needle to be guided to the tumor. The needle collects the biopsy sample and then removes it. The system goes by the name stereotaxis, or stereotactic biopsy.

The biopsy is carefully analyzed under a microscope by a pathologist, a healthcare professional specialized in diagnosing diseases through cell and tissue examination.

Chapter 4

Understanding the Grading of Brain Tumors

Brain tumors are classified on a scale of 1-4 based on their behavior, such as their growth rate and the likelihood of spreading to other parts of the brain. Over time, certain brain tumors may change their behavior, potentially progressing to a higher grade tumor or recurring as one.

Every year in the United Kingdom, around 4,300 individuals are diagnosed with slow-growing low-grade brain tumors, while 5,000 are diagnosed with fast-growing high-grade brain tumors. This amounts to a small fraction of the population in the United Kingdom.

Brain tumors are classified on a scale of 1 to 4, based on their anticipated behavior.

Tumors classified as Grade 1 and 2 (low grade)

Tumors classified as Grade 3 and 4 (high grade)

Diagnosing different types of brain tumors typically involves examining cells from the tumor obtained through a biopsy or surgery. Examining cells in the lab, a neuropathologist searches for specific cell patterns resembling different types and grades of brain tumor previously observed.

Accurate diagnosis of the grade is crucial

Getting the right diagnosis is crucial because it helps your medical team understand how the tumor might progress and suggest appropriate treatment options. This could potentially involve a clinical trial. Confirming the grade can be challenging since low-grade and high-grade tumors can appear very similar.

Low-grade brain tumors are characterized by their slow growth, well-defined edges, and low likelihood of spreading to other areas of the brain. Additionally, they have a lower chance of recurring if completely removed.

Tumors classified as Grade 1 and 2 are characterized by being low grades, slow-growing, relatively contained, and unlikely to spread to other areas of the brain. Moreover, the chances of them coming back are reduced if they can be completely eliminated. They are sometimes referred to as 'innocuous.'

These days, 'benign' is not as commonly used because it can be misleading. These less advanced brain tumors can be quite serious.

The tumor can be harmful by exerting pressure on and harming nearby areas of the brain due to the confined space within the skull. In addition, they can obstruct the flow of cerebrospinal fluid (CSF) that supports and safeguards the brain, resulting in increased pressure on the brain.

Top-Quality Tumors

High-grade brain tumors are characterized by their rapid growth, being referred to as 'malignant' or 'cancerous' growths, having a higher likelihood of spreading to other parts of the brain, and the possibility of recurring despite aggressive treatment.

Grade 3 and 4 tumors are characterized by their rapid growth and are often referred to as malignant or cancerous growths. They may extend to other regions of the brain (and, in rare cases, the spinal cord) and have the potential to recur despite aggressive treatment. Surgery alone is typically not sufficient for treatment; additional therapies like radiotherapy and chemotherapy are often necessary.

Tumors classified as 'Mixed Grade'

Various tumors consist of a mix of cells with varying levels. The tumor is classified according to the highest grade of cells it contains, even if the majority of tumor cells are low grade.

Grades of Brain Cancer

Assessing the spread of cancer beyond the original site is a crucial part of the staging process. Brain cancer is different from other types of cancer. Tumors have the ability to spread within the brain, but it is rare for primary brain tumors to metastasize outside of the brain or the Central Nervous System (CNS).

Brain cancer is typically graded instead of staged. The brain tumor grading system consists of four distinct grades. By utilizing this technique, doctors can tailor brain tumor treatments to individual requirements.

Assessing Brain Tumors

Doctors focus on examining the tumor's characteristics and its impact on various features to track brain tumor development. Key factors for assessing brain tumors are:

Dimensions and position

Types of Cells Respectability (the likelihood of being able to remove part or all of the tumor through surgery).

When cancer cells start to spread in the brain or spinal cord.

Cancer can now be found outside the brain or CNS.

Complete evaluations will also look for signs of brain cancer that are impacting vital functions, like speech, hearing, or movement.

Grading brain malignancies involves various methods that differ from staging other types of malignancies in the body. Deaths in the lungs, digestive tract, and breasts are categorized based on their position in the body, size, lymph node involvement, and potential spread.

Brain tumors are classified according to the visibility of tumor cells under a microscope.

The quality and reputation of the tumor can influence treatment choices. The success of the surgery is determined by factors such as the tumor's location, size, grade, and the patient's overall health and medical history.

Grade I (grade 1 brain tumor): The tumor typically grows at a slow pace and seldom extends into nearby tissues. Surgery could potentially remove the tumor.

Grade II brain cancers develop gradually and have the potential to spread to surrounding cells or come back.

Grade III (grade 3 brain malignancy): The tumor has the potential to multiply and spread into nearby tissue, with tumor cells appearing distinct from healthy cells.

Grade IV (grade 4 brain tumor): The tumor proliferates and metastasizes quickly, with unhealthy tumor cells.

Metastatic brain tumors are more prevalent than primary brain tumors, originating from another location in the body. As cancer treatment improves and people live longer, these tumors are increasingly common, allowing cancer to spread to the brain. Several types of cancer frequently metastasize to the brain, including lung, breast, digestive tract, kidney, melanoma, thyroid, and uterine cancers. Metastatic brain malignancy is often associated with lung malignancy. When staging lung tumors, a brain examination is typically included.

Assessment of metastatic brain cancer will be done using the Tumor, Node, Metastasized (pass on) staging system (TNM). At times, individuals may be diagnosed with a metastatic brain or vertebral tumor before discovering they have another, primary cancer.

Understanding the Origin

and Spread of Brain Tumors

A brain tumor consists of abnormal cells in the human brain. There are two main categories of brain tumors:

- Brain tumors typically originate in brain tissues and usually remain localized.

- Additional brain tumors are increasingly common. These cancers originate in a different part of the body and spread to the brain. Cancers affecting the lungs, breasts, kidneys, digestive tract, and skin are commonly known to spread to the brain.

There are brain tumors that may contain malignant cells, while others may not.

Noncancerous brain tumors do not contain cancer cells. They have a gradual development, are often removable, and rarely metastasize to neighboring brain cells. If they press on certain areas of the brain, they can lead to issues. Depending on their location in the brain, they could pose a serious risk to one's life.

Cancer cells are present in malignant brain tumors. Development rates differ, with cells having the ability to infiltrate nearby healthy brain tissues. Rarely do malignant tumors extend beyond the brain or spinal cord.

Signs of Brain Tumors

Tumors are classified based on the appearance of the cells, ranging from normal to abnormal. This measurement is crucial for your physician to plan your treatment effectively. Grading provides insight into the potential growth and spread rate of the tumor.

Grade **1:** The cells appear nearly normal and progress at a slow rate. Success in the long run is probable.

Grade 2: The cells appear slightly abnormal and progress over time. The tumor has the potential to spread to nearby tissues and may reappear later, possibly at a more severe stage.

Grade 3: The cells appear irregular and are actively proliferating near brain cells. These tumors tend to reappear.

Grade 4: The cells appear predominantly abnormal. They proliferate and disseminate rapidly.

Tumors can undergo changes. Rarely do benign tumors become cancerous, and a tumor that returns may be more aggressive.

Brain Tumor Varieties

Common types of brain cancer in adults include:

Astrocytomas typically develop in the most critical part of the brain, known as the cerebrum. They could belong to any grade level. Seizures or alterations in behavior are frequently triggered by them.

Meningiomas rank as the most prevalent primary brain tumors in adults. These are more common in your 70s or 80s. They develop in the meninges, the lining of the brain. They might fall into grades 1, 2, or 3. Typically harmless and grow slowly over time.

Oligodendrogliomas develop in the cells responsible for producing the protective covering of nerves. Grades typically range from 1 to 3. They typically have a slow growth rate and do not tend to spread to nearby tissue.

Exploring the Treatment Options for Brain Tumors

The treatment you receive will be determined by factors such as the type and stage of the tumor, its location, size, your age, and overall health.

The primary course of action typically involves surgery. Grade 1 tumors may suffice. Cancerous growths can be surgically removed, which can help reduce their size and alleviate any associated pain.

After surgery, radiation therapy can eliminate any remaining tumor cells in the area. If surgery is not an option, radiation therapy may be the only alternative.

Chemotherapy can also be utilized to eliminate cancer cells in the brain. Administered orally, intravenously, or occasionally through wafers implanted in the brain by a physician.

Specific therapy can be utilized to address particular

brain tumor types. These medications target particular components of tumor cells to halt the growth and spread of tumors. Consider asking your doctor about combined therapies as well.

Chapter 5

Therapy for Brain Cancer

The treatment for a brain tumor varies based on a variety of factors, including age, overall health, and the size, location, and type of tumor.

Both you and your family members will likely have numerous inquiries regarding brain cancers, treatment options, potential side effects, and long-term outlook. Rely on your health care and attention team for the most accurate information. Feel free to inquire.

Overview of Brain Tumor Treatment

Brain tumor treatment typically involves natural methods. Treatment programs typically consist of multiple discussions and appointments with medical professionals.

The team of doctors consists of neurosurgeons specializing in the brain and nervous system, oncologists, radiation oncologists who specialize in radiation therapy, and, naturally, most of your doctors. Consider including a dietitian, interpersonal employee, physical therapist, and potentially other specialists such as a neurologist on your team.

Procedure protocols differ significantly depending on the tumor's location, size, type, your age, and any other medical conditions you may have.

Top-notch options include surgery, radiation therapy, and chemotherapy. Typically, a variety of these can be utilized.

Brain Cancer Surgery

Surgery is a common procedure for individuals with a brain tumor.

Surgery aims to confirm the presence of a tumor identified during testing and to remove it. If the tumor cannot be removed, the surgeon will extract a sample of the tumor to identify its type.

There are cases where symptoms can be completely cured through surgery, especially with benign tumors. The neurosurgeon aims to completely remove the tumor, if feasible. Multiple treatments and procedures may be necessary prior to the surgery. As an example:

If needed, a steroid medication like dexamethasone (Decadron) may be prescribed to reduce the swelling.

You may receive anticonvulsant medication to help with or prevent seizures.

If there is an accumulation of excess cerebrospinal fluid around the brain, a shunt - a thin, plastic tube - may be inserted to help drain the fluid. The shunt is inserted into the cavity where fluid accumulates, then threaded beneath the skin to another part of the body. The fluid from the brain drains to a specific site for easy removal.

Rays Therapy for Brain Cancer

Radiotherapy, also known as rays therapy, involves using high-energy rays to eliminate tumor cells, preventing their growth and multiplication. Radiation therapy is an option for those who are not suitable candidates for surgery. After surgery, it is used to eliminate any remaining tumor cells in some cases.

Rays therapy is a specialized form of treatment. It only affects cells along its path. It generally won't harm cells in other parts of the body or in different areas of the brain.

There are various forms of radiation:

External radiation operates using a high-energy beam of radiation aimed at the tumor. As the beam travels through your skin, skull, healthy brain tissue, and other tissues, it reaches the tumor. Treatments are typically administered five times a week for a specific duration. Every treatment only takes a few minutes.

Internal or implant radiation involves using small radioactive capsules placed inside the tumor. The tablet's rays effectively eliminate the cancer cells. The tablet's radioactivity decreases gradually each day, ensuring optimal results when the ideal dosage is reached. Expect to spend several days in the hospital receiving this treatment.

This medical procedure, known as stereotactic radiosurgery, is often referred to as a "knifeless" technique, despite not involving actual surgery. It eliminates a brain tumor without the need for surgery. An imaging scan such as a CT or MRI is used to identify the exact location of the cancer in the brain. High-energy ray beams are precisely targeted at the cancer from various angles to deliver individual large doses. Rays obliterate the cancer. Stereotactic radiosurgery offers fewer complications than traditional open surgery and a quicker recovery period.

Treatment for Brain Cancer with Chemotherapy

Chemotherapy involves the use of potent medications to eliminate cancer cells.

You can use either a single medication or a combination of drugs.

Medication can be taken orally or administered intravenously. Certain medications are administered through a shunt to remove excess fluid from the brain.

Chemotherapy is typically administered in cycles. A routine involves a short period of intense treatment followed by a break for rest and recovery. Every technique has a duration of a few weeks.

Typically, regimens are designed to be completed in two to four cycles. It's important to pause and assess how your tumor has responded post-treatment.

Chemotherapy can lead to a variety of side effects. They can be challenging for many individuals to handle. Some possible side effects are nausea, vomiting, mouth sores, loss of appetite, and hair loss, among others. Some of these side effects may be alleviated or enhanced with medication.

Latest Treatments for Brain Tumors

There are constant developments in new therapies for the tumor. When a therapy demonstrates a guarantee, it undergoes analysis in a laboratory and is enhanced whenever possible. It undergoes clinical testing with individuals diagnosed with cancer.

Researchers conduct brain cancer medical trials to evaluate the effects of new medications on multiple brain cancer patients. Individuals diagnosed with brain malignancy may feel reluctant to participate in clinical trials due to fears of receiving no treatment for their condition.

There are clinical trials accessible for nearly every type of cancer. Clinical trials offer the advantage of introducing new therapies that could surpass current treatments or result in fewer side effects.

One downside is that the treatment may not be effective for everyone.

Several individuals with cancer qualify for participation in scientific trials.

Consult your oncologist for further details. The International Cancer Institute provides a concise overview of clinical tests.

After a brain tumor is diagnosed, it's important to attend all appointments with specialists and your primary care physician. Individuals with brain cancers frequently face a higher likelihood of experiencing additional health issues and potential tumor recurrence or symptom deterioration.

Success Rate of Brain Cancer Treatment

Survival rates for brain tumors can differ significantly. Several key factors influence survival rates, such as the type and location of the cancer, its operability, age, and other health conditions.

Typically, younger patients tend to have a more favorable outlook. The most common type is brain malignancy that has spread to another location in the body. Success rates hinge on the type of cancer and various other factors.

There are treatments available for certain types of brain cancers that can significantly improve your chances of survival. It's important to have a conversation with your tumor team about treatment plans and the best-estimated prognosis.

Organizations and Counseling

Dealing with cancer brings about various challenges, affecting not just you but also your loved ones. Chances are, you have numerous concerns about the impact of cancer on your daily life - from taking care of your family and home to maintaining your job and social connections. Countless individuals experience feelings of stress and depression. While some people may feel upset and resentful, others might experience feelings of helplessness and defeat.

Many individuals with cancer find it beneficial to talk about their feelings and worries.

Having a strong support system from friends and family is truly invaluable. Support may be offered once they see how you are managing. Don't wait for them to pick it up. If you have any concerns, feel free to share them.

Some people prefer not to "burden" themselves and would rather talk to a more approachable professional about their concerns. If you're looking to talk about your emotions and concerns regarding having cancer, consider reaching out to an interpersonal employee, counselor, or person in the clergy for support. Your oncologist can suggest a specialist. Speaking with others who have cancer can be incredibly beneficial for many individuals battling the disease. Sharing your worries with others who have gone through similar situations can be incredibly comforting. The American Cancers Society provides details on various cancer-related organizations across the United States.

Brain Cancer Home Care

When battling brain cancers, your healthcare team will provide details about home care to your family members. Typically, home treatment involves providing supportive measures tailored to your symptoms and individual requirements.

For example, if walking is challenging for you, physical and occupational therapists can assist in enhancing your mobility and provide tools to aid in daily tasks.

Therapeutic conversations can assist with issues concerning speech and swallowing. Home health aides have specialized training to help with personal care tasks like bathing, dressing, and eating. Home treatment may involve nurses administering medications, performing wound care, and monitoring for side effects.

When the outlook is grim, it's worth considering options such as hospice care and advance directives with medical professionals.

Home hospice care offers pain and symptom relief, along with emotional and spiritual assistance for both the patient and their family in the comfort of their own home, rather than a medical facility. It involves a diverse team of professionals such as healthcare providers, doctors, nurses, pharmacists, aides, social workers, spiritual caregivers, and counselors.

Progress directives serve as legal documents that allow you to communicate your treatment preferences and designate a decision-maker in case you become unable to do so. Various progress directives include a living will and durable power of attorney for healthcare. For example, an individual with advanced brain malignancy may choose not to undergo ventilation if they cease breathing. It is up to you to make these decisions as long as you are mentally capable.

Brain Spreading Lung Cancer

Metastasis occurs when cancer starts in one area of the body and spreads to another. When lung cancer spreads to the brain, it indicates that the original cancer has created a new tumor in the brain. Approximately 20 to 40 percent of adults diagnosed with non-small cell lung cancer develop brain metastases at some point during their illness. Common sites of metastasis include the adrenal gland, brain and nervous system, bones, liver, and lung or respiratory system.

Could you explain how lung cancer spreads to the brain?

There are two distinct forms of lung cancer:

Approximately 10 to 15 percent of lung cancers are classified as small cell lung cancer.

Non-small cell lung cancer accounts for approximately 80 to 85 percent of all lung cancers.

Lung malignancies commonly spread to other parts of the body via the lymph vessels and arteries.

Lung cancer tends to spread more easily through the lymph vessels, but it usually takes a longer time for secondary metastatic cancer to affect the lymph vessels. Arteries typically provide a tougher barrier against diseases entering the system. Once it gains momentum, it spreads rapidly.

Typically, metastasis via the bloodstream is more severe initially, while metastasis through the lymphatic system tends to have more long-term implications.

Could you please provide information on the symptoms of lung malignancy spreading to the brain?

For individuals diagnosed with lung cancer, it is crucial to pay close attention to signs of brain metastasis, such as:

Experiencing a range of symptoms like memory loss, headaches, weakness, nausea, unsteadiness, speech difficulties, numbness, tingling, and seizures.

If you experience these symptoms, it's important to notify

your doctor right away.

How to Detect Lung Cancers That Have Spread?

Doctors often rely on radiology assessments like MRI and CT scans to detect metastatic brain malignancy.

From time to time, a healthcare provider may perform a biopsy to determine the presence of brain cancer.

What is the life expectancy for lung tumors that have metastasized to the brain?

Sex, ethnicity, and age can impact survival rates, but life expectancy is typically shortened after analyzing brain metastases from lung cancer. Without any intervention, the typical success rate is less than six months from a reputable source. With proper treatment, this amount has the potential to slightly rise.

What treatments are available?

When it comes to treating lung cancer brain metastases, the options at hand are influenced by various factors, including the type of primary cancer, the number, size, and location of brain tumors, the genetic characteristics of the cancer cells, age, health status, and previous treatments.

Success Rates for Adult Brain and Spinal Cord Tumors

Survival rates provide a general idea of the outlook for individuals with a specific type of cancer. They provide information on the survival rate of people diagnosed with a similar type of tumor over a specific period, typically five years. It's impossible to predict your lifespan, but they can provide insights into the likelihood of treatment success.

What exactly does a 5-year success rate entail?

Survival rate refers to the percentage of people who survive for at least five years following their diagnosis. For example, a 5-12 months success rate of 70% indicates that around 70 out of 100 people with that type of tumor are still alive five years after diagnosis. Keep in mind that many individuals live well beyond five years.

Comparing survival rates, such as the figures provided,

offers a more precise method to gauge the impact of cancer on survival. These rates contrast individuals with the disease to the overall population. Consider this scenario: If the 5-year relative success rate for a specific type of tumor is 70%, it suggests that individuals with that tumor are typically 70% as likely as those without it to survive for at least five years post-diagnosis.

Just a reminder, the 5-season relative success rates are estimates - your perspective might vary depending on various factors unique to you.

Survival rates only provide part of the picture

Survival rates are typically determined by previous results from a significant number of individuals with the condition, but they cannot foresee the exact outcome for any specific person. It's important to consider a few limitations:

Doctors need to examine individuals who received treatment at least five years ago to determine 5-calendar year survival rates. With advancements in treatments, individuals diagnosed with brain or spinal cord tumors now have a more optimistic outlook than previously reported.

Individuals with brain or spinal cord tumors face different outlooks depending on the type of tumor and their age. Numerous factors can influence an individual's perspective, including age, overall health, tumor location, and treatment effectiveness. Each individual's perspective is shaped by their unique circumstances.

Your doctor can provide insight on how these numbers may specifically relate to you, given their knowledge of your individual circumstances.

Chapter 6

Identifying Tumor Markers and Classifications

When typical cells age or become injured, they naturally perish, making room for new cells. At times, things are not as they seem. Cells regenerate unnecessarily, while old or damaged cells linger instead of dying off. Excess cell growth can lead to the formation of masses known as tumors. Primary brain tumors range from benign to malignant.

Benign brain tumors are not made up of cancer cells. Typically, benign tumors are removable and rarely reoccur. Benign brain tumors typically display a clear border or edge. Cells from benign tumors rarely spread to surrounding tissues. They do not metastasize to other parts of your body. Yet, noncancerous growths may compress sensitive parts of the brain, leading to significant health problems.

Benign brain tumors, unlike those in most other parts of the body, can sometimes be life-threatening. There is a possibility for benign brain tumors to transform into malignant ones.

Brain cancer, or malignant brain tumors, are a serious threat as they tend to grow and invade nearby healthy brain tissue. Cancer cells from these tumors can break off and spread to other parts of the brain or the spinal cord, although they typically do not spread to other areas of the body.

Grade of the Tumor

Doctors categorize brain tumors based on their grade. The tumor standard determines the types of cells that will be observed under a microscope.

Grade I: The cells are noncancerous. These cells resemble healthy brain cells and have a slow growth rate.

Grade II: The tissues are cancerous. The cells resemble

those found in a Grade I tumor more than healthy cells.

Grade III: The cancerous cells exhibit a distinct difference in appearance compared to normal cells. The irregular cells are displaying positive growth (anaplastic).

Grade IV: The cancerous cells appear highly abnormal and have a strong tendency to divide rapidly.

Cells from low-grade tumors (grades I and II) appear more typical and tend to progress at a slower pace compared to cells from high-grade tumors (grades III and IV).

Over time, a low-grade tumor may progress to a high-grade tumor. Yet, the transition to a high-grade tumor occurs more frequently in adults than in children.

Major Brain Tumor Categories

Primary brain tumors come in different types. Among adults, the most common types of brain tumors include astrocytoma, oligodendroglioma, and meningioma.

Brain tumors are classified according to the type of cells

or the specific region of the brain where they originate. For example, the majority of primary brain tumors originate in glial cells. This particular type of tumor is known as a glioma.

Gliomas originate from glial cells found in the supportive cells of the brain. Various types of gliomas are categorized based on their location and the origin of the tumor. Here are some types of gliomas:

- Astrocytoma originates from star-shaped glial cells known as astrocytes. It has the potential to be any grade. Among adults, an astrocytoma commonly develops in the cerebrum.

- Known as a low-grade glioma, a Grade I or II astrocytoma is a possibility.

- Grade III astrocytoma is also known as a high-grade or anaplastic astrocytoma.

- Grade IV astrocytoma is also known as glioblastoma (GBM) or malignant astrocytic glioma.

Oligodendroglioma: This tumor originates from cells that generate the fatty material protecting nerves. Typically found in the cerebrum. Typically seen in individuals in their middle years. It might be classified as either grade II or III.

Meningiomas typically grow slowly and are noncancerous tumors that develop from the membranes covering the brain just beneath the skull. This type of tumor accounts for approximately one-third of brain tumors in adults. A tumor has developed in the meninges. It might fall under grades I, II, or III. Typically, it is considered benign (grade I) and grows at a slow pace.

When it comes to children, the most common types of tumors include:

- Medulloblastoma typically develops in the cerebellum. It's also known as a primitive neuroectodermal tumor. It's classified as grade IV.

- Low-grade astrocytoma can develop anywhere in the brain in children. One of the most common types of astrocytoma in children is the juvenile pilocytic astrocytoma. This is a Grade I.

- Ependymoma The tumor originates from cells that have accumulated at the ventricles or the central canal of the spinal cord. It primarily affects children and adults. Grades could range from I to III.

Brainstem glioma: This tumor develops in a prominent region of the brain. It can be either a low-grade or high-grade tumor. One common type is diffuse intrinsic pontine glioma.

Understanding Brain Tumor Levels and Prognostic Factors

For various types of tumors in different parts of the body, a staging system is used to indicate the tumor's location, spread, and impact on other body parts. There is no established systemic staging system for adult brain tumors since primary tumors typically do not spread beyond the Central Nervous System. The grading system detailed below is consistently utilized as it determines the specific characteristics of a brain tumor, influencing its malignancy and growth potential.

Factors for Predicting Outcomes

Identifying the most suitable treatment for a brain tumor involves determining both the type and grade of the tumor. Several factors contribute to doctors' understanding of the appropriate brain tumor treatment and a patient's prognosis:

Examining the histology of the tumor

As detailed in the Analysis section, a tumor sample is extracted for assessment. Tumor histology encompasses the type of tumor, its grade, and additional molecular characteristics that can predict its growth rate. Together, these factors can assist your doctor in understanding how the tumor will act. These factors play a crucial role in shaping a patient's treatment plans.

Grades indicate particular characteristics in the tumor linked to specific outcomes. Doctors may assess whether the tumor cells are proliferating rapidly or if there is a notable presence of deceased cells. Tumors displaying characteristics typically linked with rapid growth are assigned a higher grade. With certain tumors, a lower grade often indicates a more favorable prognosis.

Glial tumors are graded according to their microscopic features using specific criteria.

Grade I tumors grow slowly and are unlikely to spread. Surgery is frequently used for their treatment.

Grade II tumors have a lower tendency to spread but tend to recur despite treatment.

Grade III tumors consist of rapidly dividing cells without any dead cells. They have the ability to reproduce rapidly.

Grade IV tumors have rapidly dividing cells within them. Moreover, the tumor exhibits blood vessel growth and areas of necrotic tissue. These tumors have the potential to grow and spread rapidly.

Age Bracket

When diagnosing adults, considering the individual's age

group and functional position can be key in predicting the patient's prognosis. In most cases, a younger adult tends to have a more positive outlook.

Signs and symptoms

Symptoms and their duration can also play a role in determining prognosis. For example, experiencing seizures and having symptoms for a prolonged period are linked to a more positive outlook.

Tumor Residual Degree of Resection involves surgically removing a tumor. A patient's chances of recovery significantly improve when all tumors can be surgically removed. Here are four classifications:

Total amount: The tumor has been completely removed. Nevertheless, tiny cells might remain.

Subtotal: Significant portions of the tumor have been extracted.

Only a portion of the tumor is removed.

Biopsy exclusive: Just a small portion is taken for a

biopsy.

Location of the Tumor

Tumors have the potential to form in various regions of the brain. Certain tumor locations can be more detrimental, and treating tumors in certain locations can be more challenging.

Characteristics at the molecular level

Specific genetic mutations in the tumor can play a role in predicting the outcome. Among these are: IDH1, IDH2, MGMT, and a 1p/19q co-deletion. At times, the presence of these mutations can influence the type of brain tumor that is identified.

Neurological Functioning

The doctor will evaluate an individual's ability to function and carry out daily activities using a practical assessment scale, such as the Karnofsky Performance Scale (KPS), described below. A higher score signifies an improved functional status. Generally, individuals who can walk and care for themselves tend to have a more positive outlook.

- 100 No issues, no evidence of illness

- 90 Able to maintain regular activities; minor disease symptoms

- 80 Able to work normally; experiencing some disease symptoms

- 70 Self-care possible; unable to engage in normal activities or strenuous work

- 60 Needs occasional help but can manage personal needs

- 50 Needs significant and regular aid and health care

- 40 Disabled: needs specialized care and assistance

- 30 Severely disabled individuals may require hospitalization, although their condition is not immediately life-threatening. Those who are very ill should be hospitalized and receive vigorous treatment. Declining, critical functions advancing swiftly

Metastatic Spread out

If a tumor originates in the brain or spinal cord and is cancerous, it typically does not spread to other parts of the body in adults. However, it may continue to grow within the central nervous system. Therefore, in most cases, tests examining other organs in your body are usually unnecessary. When a tumor spreads to other parts of the brain or spinal cord, the outlook is usually not as good.

Tumor that keeps coming back

A recurrent tumor is one that continues to reappear following treatment. In case the tumor comes back, further examinations will be necessary to determine the extent of the recurrence. These scans are similar to the ones conducted during the initial analysis.

Currently, the elements listed above will serve as the most reliable indicators of the patient's prognosis. Experts are currently searching for biomarkers in tumor cells to facilitate the diagnosis of brain tumors, as discussed in Diagnosis. Researchers are exploring additional genetic tests that could potentially forecast a patient's outlook. In the future, these tools could assist doctors in predicting the growth of brain tumors, improving treatments, and forecasting prognosis more accurately.

Chapter 7

Glomeromatoma: What is it?

Glioblastoma is a type of brain cancer. This is the most common type of cancerous brain tumor in adults. It's typically quite intense, leading to rapid development and quick spread. While a permanent solution is not available, there are therapies that can provide relief from symptoms.

Where does it originate in the brain?

Glioblastoma, a type of astrocytoma, is a malignant tumor that originates from star-shaped cells in the brain known as astrocytes. Typically, this cancer originates in the cerebrum, the most crucial region of the human brain, in adults.

Glioblastoma tumors enhance their blood circulation to support their growth. These can potentially infiltrate healthy brain tissues.

How prevalent is it?

Brain tumors are not frequently seen. When they happen, approximately 80% are not glioblastomas. Men are more likely to have them than women. Opportunities increase as you get older. Around 14,000 cases of glioblastoma are diagnosed in the U.S. annually by doctors.

Symptoms Glioblastomas typically lead to the first symptoms due to their rapid multiplication and the strain they put on the brain. If the tumor is located in a specific area, it may lead to a range of symptoms such as persistent headaches, seizures, vomiting, cognitive difficulties, alterations in mood or behavior, vision problems, and speech impairments.

Diagnosis

Get ready for a thorough medical examination by a neurologist, a specialist in brain disorders. You have the option to undergo an MRI or CT scan, as well as other examinations, based on your symptoms.

Glioblastoma treatment aims to decelerate and manage tumor growth. It assists in making you feel as comfortable as possible. There are four treatments available, and it's common for individuals to receive multiple kinds.

The initial course of action involves surgery. The doctor aims to remove as much of the tumor as feasible. It may not always be feasible to completely eliminate all elements in critical areas of the brain.

Utilizing radiation helps eliminate any remaining tumor cells post-surgery. Moreover, it could potentially impede the growth of tumors that are inoperable.

Chemotherapy can also be beneficial. Temozolomide stands out as the standard chemotherapy drug prescribed by doctors for glioblastoma. Chemotherapy may result in temporary side effects, but it is much less damaging than in the past.

Physicians have the ability to address glioblastoma that returns by using another chemotherapy drug known as carmustine (or BCNU). Electric field therapy targets tumor cells specifically, without causing harm to healthy cells. Doctors place electrodes on the head to complete this procedure. This device goes by the name Optune. It is acquired through chemotherapy following surgery and radiation treatment. It has been approved by the FDA for individuals who have been recently diagnosed and those whose glioblastoma has recurred.

Major cancer-treatment centers offer access to experimental treatments, including dental chemotherapy that can be administered at home. These treatments may alleviate symptoms and potentially shrink the tumor in some individuals.

Glioblastomas have a tendency to recur. If this situation arises, physicians could potentially treat it through surgical procedures and alternative radiation and chemotherapy methods. Palliative care is essential for individuals dealing with a serious illness. It aims to alleviate cancer symptoms in order to improve your quality of life. Consider consulting your doctor about potential clinical trials that could be suitable for you.

Outlook and Rates of Success

Several factors impact a person's outcome when dealing with cancer, such as glioblastomas. It's difficult for doctors to predict a person's life expectancy with a glioblastoma. They possess data that monitors the typical outcomes for different cancer sizes among individuals who have faced these conditions over time.

When it comes to glioblastoma, here are the success rates:

- Twelve months: 40.2%

- 2 years: 17.4%

- Over a span of five years, the percentage increase was 5.6.

Numbers cannot accurately forecast an individual's future. Age group, type of tumor, and overall health all play a role in this. With advancements in treatments, individuals newly diagnosed with these aggressive brain tumors may experience significantly improved results.

What is the significance of Grade 4 Astrocytoma?

Glioblastomas are sometimes referred to as grade 4 astrocytoma tumors. Tumors are classified on a scale from 1 to 4 based on their degree of deviation from normal cells. The grade indicates the speed at which the tumor is likely to grow and spread. Grade 4 tumors are known for their aggressive nature and rapid growth. It has a rapid spread.

Categories of Glioblastoma

There are two types of glioblastoma that you can find:

- De novo glioblastoma is the most common type of this cancer. This is also the most extreme form.

- Supplementary glioblastoma is a rare type of tumor that tends to grow at a slower pace. Typically, it starts with a lower-grade, less aggressive astrocytoma, with secondary glioblastoma affecting around ten percent of people with this type of brain cancer. Many individuals familiar with this type of cancer are aged 45 or younger.

Glioblastomas typically develop in the frontal and temporal lobes of the brain. These can also be located in the brain stem, cerebellum, other regions of the brain, and the spinal cord.

Survival rates and life expectancy

Individuals with glioblastoma typically have a median survival time of 15 to 16 months when they undergo surgery, chemotherapy, and radiation therapy. Half of the patients with this tumor survive until the specified time.

Each individual with glioblastoma is unique. Some people have a short lifespan. Some individuals can endure for up to five years or even longer, though it is rare.

Among children, those with higher-grade tumors typically have a longer survival rate compared to adults. Approximately a quarter of children diagnosed with this tumor survive for five years or longer.

Increasing longevity

Exciting advancements in treatments are further increasing life expectancy. Individuals with tumors that possess a strong hereditary marker known as MGMT methylation tend to have higher success rates.

MGMT functions to preserve cells that have been harmed. Chemotherapy eradicates glioblastoma cells, while MGMT repairs them. MGMT methylation plays a crucial role in inhibiting repair mechanisms, leading to increased destruction of tumor cells.

Treatments for Glioblastoma

Glioblastoma can be challenging to manage. Rapidly increasing, these projections extend into the healthy brain, posing challenges for surgical removal. These tumors are composed of various cell types. Certain treatments may be highly effective on certain cells, but not on others.

Glioblastoma treatment typically includes surgery to remove as much of the tumor as feasible.

- Radiation treatment to eliminate any remaining tumor cells post-surgery

- Chemotherapy using the drug temozolomide (temodar)

Additional medications that can be utilized to treat this cancer are:

- Bevacizumab (Avastin)

- Polifeprosan 20 with carmustine implant (Gliadel)

- Lomustine (Ceenu).

Exciting new treatments for glioblastoma are currently under evaluation in clinical trials. The following treatments are included:

- Utilizing your body's natural disease-fighting ability to eliminate cancer cells is the concept behind immunotherapy.

- Gene therapy involves fixing faulty genes to combat cancer.

- Utilizing stem cells, known as primitive cells, for cancer treatment.

- Enhance your body's ability to fight cancer with Vaccine Therapy.

- Personalized Medicine, also referred to as targeted therapy.

If approved, these treatments and others have the potential to significantly improve the complete recovery of individuals with glioblastoma in the future.

Causes and Risk Factors

Physicians are not entirely sure about the cause of glioblastoma. Similar to other cancers, it initiates when cells begin to proliferate uncontrollably, leading to the formation of tumors. Men are at a higher risk of developing this type of tumor.

- Aged 50 and over.

- Caucasian or Asian descent.

Symptoms of Glioblastoma

When glioblastoma puts pressure on certain parts of the brain, symptoms may appear. When the tumor is small, you may not experience any noticeable symptoms. The symptoms you experience vary based on the location of the tumor in the brain.

Here are some symptoms to look out for: headaches,

nausea and vomiting, sleepiness, weakness in one part of the body, memory loss, speech and language difficulties, changes in personality, muscle weakness, double or blurry vision, loss of appetite, and seizures.

Chapter 8

When is it advisable to seek medical attention for a brain tumor?

If you experience the following symptoms, it's crucial to seek treatment from a physician right away, possibly urgently:

- Experiencing persistent vomiting without a clear cause.

- Experiencing sudden changes in vision, such as unexplained blurriness on one side.

- Feeling tired or more sleepy than usual.

- Experiencing new seizures.

- Experiencing a new type of headache, particularly in the morning hours.

Headaches are a common symptom of brain cancer, but they may not manifest until later stages of the condition. If there is a sudden and significant change in someone's headache pattern, healthcare professionals may recommend visiting the diagnosis department. If someone has a known brain tumor, experiencing new symptoms, sudden worsening of symptoms, or unexpected changes should prompt a visit to the nearest emergency department. Keep an eye out for upcoming indicators:

- Experiencing seizures.

- Mental shifts like increased drowsiness or difficulty focusing.

- Noticing visible changes or experiencing sensory issues.

- Struggling with communication or articulation.

- Behavior or personality alterations.

- Experiencing clumsiness or challenges with walking.

- Experience nausea and vomiting, particularly in middle-aged or elderly individuals.

- When a fever appears suddenly, especially in someone undergoing chemotherapy.

Can Examinations and Tests Diagnose Brain Cancer?

If symptoms arise suddenly, many individuals may undergo a brain CT scan. This test is akin to an X-ray but provides more detailed information in three dimensions.

Typically, a dye, referred to as a contrast material, is injected into the bloodstream to emphasize any abnormalities on the scan. Individuals with brain cancer often experience additional medical issues, leading to the need for routine laboratory tests.

These include examining blood, electrolyte levels, liver function, and blood clotting.

When mental-status change is the initial sign, blood or urine tests may be conducted to rule out drug use as a potential cause of the symptoms. One common method to assess the type and size of a brain tumor is through an MRI scan. It's important to note that not all hospitals have MRI scanners available.

One reason for this is that MRI is more sensitive in detecting the presence and features of the tumor. Examining the connection between cancer and the surrounding brain, including brain coverings, cerebrospinal fluid spaces, and vascular structures, helps in making a preliminary diagnosis of the tumor.

Currently, though, numerous institutions with MRI scanners continue to rely on CT scans for tumor screening.

If CT or MRI scans reveal the presence of a brain tumor, the person will likely be recommended to undergo brain surgery by a team of specialists including a neurosurgeon, radiation oncologist, and possibly a medical oncologist specializing in chemotherapy for brain tumors.

Confirming whether the individual has brain cancer is the next step in the diagnosis process. Viewing a scan may raise doubts about the presence of a brain tumor, but confirming it depends on getting a cell diagnosis whenever possible. A biopsy is performed to determine the type and stage of the tumor.

One of the most effective methods for locating a biopsy is through a medical procedure known as a craniotomy. The skull is typically opened to completely remove the tumor, if feasible. An extraction is performed to obtain a biopsy from the tumor.

If the doctor has difficulty extracting the entire tumor, a portion of the cancer is eliminated. There are cases where a biopsy can be performed without the need to open the skull. The tumor's exact location in the brain is determined using CT or MRI scans while the brain remains stationary in a framework. A small opening is carefully made in the skull, allowing a needle to reach the tumor. The needle collects the biopsy sample and removes it. The system is known as stereotaxis, or stereotactic biopsy. This method is not aimed at curing the tumor but is usually used when the tumor is hard to reach or responds well to radiation therapy (like CNS lymphoma or pineal germ cell tumor), and surgery is not necessary for effective treatment.

The biopsy is analyzed under a microscope by a pathologist (the physician specializing in diagnosing diseases by examining cells and tissues) and typically given an NCI grade.

What treatments are available for brain cancer?

Customized treatment plans are essential for patients with brain cancers. Treatment programs are tailored to the patient's age group, health status, tumor characteristics, and other relevant factors. Typically, surgery, radiation, and chemotherapy are the main treatment options for brain cancer. There are various treatment options available. Below, we will delve into the different types of procedures.

People close to the patient may have numerous inquiries regarding the tumor, the procedure, the impact of treatment, and the long-term prognosis. Consulting with the individual's healthcare team is the most effective way to acquire this information. Feel free to ask if you have any more questions.

Brain Cancer Self-Care

It is important for the person's doctor and the physician team in charge of their case to communicate details about home care with both the patient and their family.

Typically, home treatment involves providing necessary support tailored to the patient's symptoms. When mental status changes occur, it's important to tailor the care plan to meet the patient's specific needs. For example, a nurse might be assigned to oversee the patient's daily medications.

When the patient's prognosis is not favorable, discussing hospice care and advance directives with the doctors is appropriate.

Home hospice care offers pain and symptom relief, along with emotional and spiritual support for both the individual and their family, in the comfort of their own home instead of a medical facility. A multidisciplinary approach involving various healthcare professionals such as physicians, nurses, pharmacists, aides, social workers, religious caregivers, and counselors is necessary.

Legal documents known as progress directives and living wills specify which treatments to administer and which to refrain from. Consider this scenario: someone diagnosed with an advanced brain tumor may choose not to use a ventilator if they stop breathing. Patients are entitled to make these decisions independently as long as they remain mentally competent. Healthcare personnel must have easy access to directives, especially when there is a sudden change in the individual's condition. Otherwise, the person's treatment directives may not be followed.

There are various home remedies for brain cancer available online, from folic acid supplements to antioxidants and natural substances. There is minimal data to support these claims, so it's important for patients to discuss these treatments with their doctors before trying them.

Medical Procedure Programs for Brain Cancer

Procedure protocols differ significantly depending on the tumor's location, size, grade, and type, the patient's age, and any other medical conditions the individual may have.

Top-notch treatments include surgery, radiation therapy, and chemotherapy. Some treatment types can be utilized in various situations. Surgery is a common procedure for many individuals with brain tumors. Craniotomy is the term for the surgical opening of the skull.

Surgery aims to confirm the nature of the abnormality observed on the brain scan, determine the tumor's grade, and remove the tumor. If the tumor cannot be eliminated, the doctor will conduct a test on the tumor to identify its type and grade.

There are cases where surgery can completely cure the condition, especially with benign tumors. If feasible, a neurosurgeon will attempt to remove the tumor.

Patients often experience various treatments and approaches before resorting to surgery. A steroid medication like dexamethasone (Decadron) could be prescribed to reduce the swelling.

Anticonvulsant medication like levetiracetam (Keppra), phenytoin (Dilantin), or carbamazepine (Tegretol) may be prescribed to help with seizures.

Overview of Brain Tumor Resection Surgery

The goal of tumor surgery is to remove as much of the tumor as safely achievable while minimizing the impact on brain function. Patients at the highest level undergo this procedure while under general anesthesia. Certain surgeries are performed while the patient is awake or under light sedation to map vocabulary function. When undergoing surgery with general anesthesia, a tube is inserted into the windpipe. However, for surgeries performed while awake, a mask is used to help with breathing and the person is sedated. The head is positioned securely with a clamp system to prevent any movement of the skull. An image-guided navigation system is frequently utilized to precisely identify the exact location of the incision. First, the head is prepared, then the mouth is clipped. Next, the incision area is infiltrated with local anesthesia, and the head is incised to expose the skull bone. Part of the skulls are delicately cut open, revealing the inner tissues of the brain. When it's crucial to assess potential brain function impairment, the person is roused from sedation to respond while mapping techniques are carried out.

After all, the tumor resection is then finalized. Tumors are typically sent to a pathologist for assessment. One option for the surgeon is to insert biodegradable polymer wafers containing chemotherapy drugs (Gliadel wafers) into the tumor cavity. Once the tumor resection is finished, the brain's surrounding membranes are closed, and the skull is typically sealed with titanium plates and screws to maintain its position. After the procedure, some cosmetic surgeons may place drains under the head for a day or two to minimize the accumulation of blood or fluid.

Using stereotactic radiosurgery, a modern technique eliminates a brain tumor without the need to open the skull. A CT or MRI scan is used to identify the exact location of the tumor in the brain. The tumor affects high-energy radiation beams from various angles. Rays eliminate the tumor. Gamma blades utilize concentrated gamma rays, linear accelerators use photons, and heavy-charged particle radiosurgery operates on the proton beam.

Knifeless procedures offer fewer complications and a significantly shorter recovery time. Drawbacks include the limited availability of cells for pathology analysis and potential brain swelling following radiation treatment.

If a tumor causes a blockage in the fluid passageways, a shunt - a thin plastic tube - may be inserted to drain the excess cerebrospinal fluid buildup. One end of the shunt is positioned in the cavity where fluid accumulates, while the other end is inserted under the skin to a different part of the body. This allows the fluid to flow from the brain to a specific site where it can be effortlessly extracted.

Brain Tumors that cannot be operated on

Tumors that are considered inoperable are located in a part of the brain that surgeons cannot access. However, even if the doctors can access the tumor, they may have to remove or damage a significant amount of surrounding brain tissue, potentially causing harm to the patient equal to that of the tumor. Tumors, regardless of type or size, may be inoperable. If a doctor is confident they can access the tumor without disturbing critical brain functions like speech or movement, then the tumor is considered operable. Some tumors are deemed inoperable when arteries penetrate them to a degree where removing the tumor and its vascular system would likely result in severe harm or death to the patient. When a surgeon deems a patient's brain tumor inoperable, seeking a second opinion from another physician is advisable. Another doctor might have a different perspective and consider the tumor to be "operable." In such cases, doctors may opt for Whole-Brain Rays' Therapy (WBRT) to treat inoperable brain tumors gradually over several weeks.

Exploring Rays, Chemotherapy, and Clinical Tests for Brain Cancer

Radiotherapy, also known as rays therapy, involves using high-energy rays to eliminate tumor cells and prevent their growth and multiplication.

For some individuals, radiation therapy may be an alternative when surgery is not an option. After surgery, it can also be utilized to eradicate any remaining tumor cells. Tomotherapy, which involves modulated rays therapy aided by CT checking, can also be utilized.

Rays therapy targets specific cells along its path, providing localized treatment. It typically doesn't harm cells in other parts of the body or in other areas of the brain.

Rays can be given in two different ways:

External radiation operates using a high-energy beam of radiation aimed at the tumor. The beam travels through your skin, skull, healthy brain tissue, and other cells to reach the tumor. Treatments are typically administered five times a week for about 4-6 weeks. Every session will only last a few minutes. Two techniques, the gamma blade and cyber blade, involve using external radiation to eliminate cancer cells in the brain.

Internal or implant radiation involves a small radioactive capsule placed directly inside the tumor. The cancer is eradicated by the rays emitted from the capsule. Each day, the tablet's radioactivity decreases slightly as the radiation amount is precisely calculated to determine the ideal dosage. Patients need to be in a healthcare facility for a few days to receive this treatment.

Chemotherapy involves the use of potent medications to eliminate cancer cells. You have the option to use either a single medication or a combination of medications. Previous treatments for brain cancers involved medications such as BCNU and CCNU, procarbazine, and vincristine. There are different ways of administering medication: orally or through intravenous injection.

Two medications, temozolomide (Temodar) and bevacizumab (Avastin), have been authorized for treating malignant gliomas. New medications might enhance productivity and have fewer side effects than older ones. One of the advantages of Temozolomide is that it can be taken by mouth, removing the need for IV lines and hospital stays for chemotherapy.

Chemotherapy is typically administered in cycles. A routine involves a short period of intense treatment followed by a break for rest and recovery. Every technique has a duration of a few weeks.

Typically, regimens are designed to be completed in two to four cycles. There appears to be a disruption in the process, and scans are conducted to assess the tumor's response to prompt treatment.

Chemotherapy side effects are now more manageable and easier to endure. Some common side effects are nausea, vomiting, mouth sores, loss of appetite, hair loss, and others. Some of these side effects can be alleviated or enhanced with medication.

Novel treatments such as utilizing nanotechnology to deliver medication directly to cancer cells are continuously being created. When research therapy demonstrates potential, it undergoes examination in laboratories for enhancement. People with cancer are often observed through scientific trials.

Clinical trials offer the advantage of introducing new therapies that could surpass current treatments or result in fewer side effects. Several individuals with cancer qualify for participation in medical trials.

Consult a healthcare professional for further details. The website of the National Cancer Institute provides a summary of scientific trials.

Various treatments for brain tumors are mentioned in websites, health magazines, and other publications, such as Transfer Factor, Cellect, and Vitalzym. Several products lack medical data to support their claims. Visitors are advised to carefully read the fine print on these websites as many state that the products are not intended to cure specific illnesses. It's important for patients to consult their doctors before purchasing and using such substances. According to the FDA, certain health supplements are not considered active or safe.

Side Effects of Brain Cancer Treatments

Treatment plans aim to minimize or alleviate side effects linked to brain cancer treatment. Nevertheless, the majority of patients may encounter certain side effects, with some being quite severe. People undergoing brain tumor treatment should inquire about potential side effects, evaluate the benefits of the recommended treatment, and plan for managing any side effects that may arise.

Chemotherapy may lead to side effects such as nausea, vomiting, hair loss, and fatigue. When the immune system is weakened, it can leave a person more susceptible to illnesses. Additional organ systems such as the kidneys or reproductive organs may be affected. While these side effects usually diminish after treatment, some may persist, especially if other organ systems are affected.

Radiation therapy produces similar outcomes to chemotherapy, but with potentially fewer side effects since it doesn't directly expose multiple organ systems to radiation. Nevertheless, skin may experience surface damage such as reddish or darkened areas, along with increased sensitivity. Thinning of the hair may occur in regions exposed to sunlight, and in some cases, it can be permanent.

Undergoing surgery can lead to various effects, including short-term and long-term changes. Some of these effects may include brain swelling and damage to healthy cells. Changes in mental status, muscle weakness, or alterations in various brain-controlled functions may manifest. While most side effects tend to diminish over time, there is a possibility that some may be long-lasting.

Patients and individuals with brain cancers should carefully evaluate potential side effects, as some may be mitigated through treatment and not necessarily permanent. Patients with brain malignancy seeking treatment need to be aware that without surgery, chemotherapy, or radiation therapy (or combinations of these), the outlook for some patients is not favorable.

Brain Cancer Check-up

After a brain tumor is diagnosed, it's crucial for the

person to attend all appointments with consultants and the main doctor. Typically, individuals with brain cancer face a higher likelihood of experiencing additional health issues and potential symptom relapse or deterioration. It's important to ask doctors for survivor treatment plans that outline past treatments and recommendations for follow-up care and managing indicators.

After treatment, patients will schedule follow-up visits with their cancer care team. Regular follow-up checkups and examinations will be recommended. This follow-up aims to promptly identify any tumor recurrence or long-term effects of the procedure for immediate treatment.

Ways to prevent brain cancer

Typically, there is no proven method to prevent brain malignancies. Yet, by implementing new analysis and treatment methods for tumors that have a tendency to spread to the brain, the risk of metastatic brain tumors could be reduced. Avoiding exposure to radiation, toxic chemicals from the oil and rubber industry, embalming chemicals, and other environmental toxins can reduce the risk of developing brain cancers. It is also recommended to prevent HIV infection.

According to popular sources and various websites, refraining from using mobile phones and following a macrobiotic diet may reduce the risk of brain cancer. Currently, there is no concrete evidence to support these claims. A study conducted in December 2010, involving approximately 59,000 mobile phone users with usage spanning from five to ten years, concluded that there was no significant increase in brain cancer rates among them. Investigators claim that prolonged use of mobile phones has not been thoroughly examined. In 2016, the National Cancer Institute released results from multiple studies that compiled findings, with the majority indicating no link between cancer and mobile phone usage. For those looking to minimize radiation exposure from mobile phones, they can find a list online detailing phones with the lowest radiation levels.

What is the outlook for a brain tumor?

What is the life expectancy for someone with brain

cancer?

Several key factors impact brain cancer survival, including the type of cancer, its location, the possibility of surgical intervention, and the overall health of the person.

The long-term survival rate for individuals with primary brain cancer can vary. For severe cases of advanced brain tumors, the survival rate ranges from less than 10% to around 32%, even with aggressive surgery, radiation, and chemotherapy.

Treatments can extend survival in the short term and also enhance quality of life for a considerable period, although the duration may vary.

Post-surgery, exposure to rays can significantly improve a patient's chances of success compared to not receiving treatment at all. Chemotherapy can extend life for some patients when administered in conjunction with radiation therapy.

People with persistent seizures that are hard to control

even with medication tend to have a poor outcome in the following six months. It's important to have a conversation with the patient's cancer team about treatment plans and the best-estimated prognosis.

Organizations, Resources, and Support for Brain Cancer Patients

Dealing with cancer brings about various challenges for the person affected, as well as their loved ones. Patients often have concerns about how cancer will impact their ability to maintain a normal life, including taking care of family and home, continuing with work, and sustaining friendships and activities.

Countless individuals experience feelings of stress and depression. Some people experience intense anger and bitterness, while others may feel powerless and defeated. Discussing their emotions and concerns can be beneficial for many individuals dealing with cancer.

Family and friends are often a great source of support. Support may be withheld until the person's response to the condition is observed. If patients wish to address their concerns, they should feel inspired to seek support from their family and friends.

Some people prefer not to "burden" themselves and would rather talk about their concerns with a more approachable professional. Seeking support from a social worker, counselor, or member of the clergy can be beneficial for individuals looking to discuss their emotions and worries related to cancer. Your oncologist can suggest a suitable specialist. During a difficult time, hospice can provide valuable support for both patients with terminal cancer and their family members.

Speaking with others who have cancer can be incredibly beneficial for many individuals battling the disease. Connecting with individuals who have gone through a similar experience can provide a great sense of comfort. You may find groups of people with similar conditions at the hospital where you are receiving treatment. The American Malignancy Society provides details about additional pertinent organizations across the United States.

Acknowledgements

Behold the magnificent triumph of this extraordinary book, a testament to the divine intervention of God Almighty and the unwavering love and support of my cherished Family, devoted Fans, avid Readers, loyal Customers, and dear Friends. Their ceaseless encouragement has paved the way for this resounding success.

www.ingramcontent.com/pod-product-compliance
Lightning Source LLC
Chambersburg PA
CBHW031130020426
42333CB00012B/306